DR. BARBARA MUCUS CLEANSE

Revitalize your health: Dr. Barbara's proven mucus cleanse-discover effective methods to clear your system, boost immunity and reclaim vitality

Miguel Sofia

Table of Contents

COPYRIGHT © 2023

CHAPTER ONE

Introduction to Dr. Barbara's Approach to Herbal Healing and Mucus Cleanse

Dr. Barbara's approach to herbal healing and mucus cleanse is founded on the principles of holistic health, natural remedies, and traditional herbalism. It encompasses a comprehensive understanding of the body's systems, the role of herbs in promoting wellness, and the importance of addressing underlying imbalances to achieve optimal health. In this detailed exploration, we'll delve into the fundamental concepts, methodologies, and benefits of Dr. Barbara's approach to herbal healing and mucus cleanse.

Understanding Herbal Healing

Herbal healing is a practice that dates back thousands of years, rooted in various cultures worldwide. It involves the use of plants and plant extracts to promote health, prevent illness, and alleviate symptoms. Dr. Barbara's approach to herbal healing emphasizes the potency and efficacy of botanical remedies in supporting the body's innate healing mechanisms.

Central to this approach is the recognition that plants contain a wealth of bioactive compounds, including vitamins, minerals, antioxidants, and phytochemicals, which exert therapeutic effects on the body. These compounds interact with physiological processes, modulating inflammation, supporting immune function, and promoting overall well-being. By harnessing the healing power of herbs, individuals can address a wide range of health concerns while minimizing the risk of adverse effects associated with synthetic medications.

The Importance of Mucus Cleanse

Mucus cleanse, also known as mucus elimination or detoxification, is a crucial aspect of Dr. Barbara's approach to health and wellness. The human body produces mucus as a protective mechanism, lining the respiratory tract, gastrointestinal tract, and other mucous membranes to trap pathogens, dust, and other foreign particles. However, excessive mucus production or impaired mucus clearance can lead to congestion, inflammation, and susceptibility to infections.

A mucus cleanse aims to support the body's natural detoxification pathways, facilitating the expulsion of excess mucus and promoting respiratory and gastrointestinal health. This process involves various strategies, including dietary modifications, hydration, herbal remedies, and lifestyle changes. By clearing excess mucus from the body, individuals can experience improved breathing, enhanced digestion, and a greater sense of vitality.

Key Concepts in Dr. Barbara's Approach

Dr. Barbara's approach to herbal healing and mucus cleanse revolves around several key concepts that guide her practice and recommendations:

1. **Holistic Health**: Dr. Barbara views health as a multifaceted interplay of physical, emotional, and spiritual well-being. Her approach considers the interconnectedness of body, mind, and spirit, recognizing that imbalances in one aspect can manifest as symptoms in others. By addressing the root causes of illness and supporting the body as a whole, she promotes holistic healing and long-term wellness.

2. **Individualized Care**: Each person is unique, with distinct health needs, genetic predispositions, and lifestyle factors. Dr. Barbara's approach emphasizes personalized care, tailoring herbal remedies and treatment plans to suit the individual's specific constitution and health goals. This individualized approach ensures optimal outcomes and enhances the efficacy of herbal healing and mucus cleanse protocols.

3. **Natural Remedies**: Nature provides a vast array of healing substances, from medicinal herbs and botanical extracts to wholesome foods and therapeutic practices. Dr. Barbara advocates for the use of natural remedies that work in harmony with the body's innate wisdom, avoiding harsh

chemicals and synthetic compounds whenever possible. By harnessing the healing power of nature, individuals can support their health naturally and sustainably.

4. **Gentle Detoxification**: Detoxification is a natural process through which the body eliminates toxins and metabolic waste products. Dr. Barbara's approach to mucus cleanse emphasizes gentle detoxification methods that support the body's detox pathways without causing undue stress or discomfort. This may include herbal teas, dietary changes, hydrotherapy, and lifestyle modifications designed to enhance detoxification and promote overall health.

Benefits of Dr. Barbara's Approach

The holistic approach to herbal healing and mucus cleanse advocated by Dr. Barbara offers a wide range of benefits for individuals seeking to optimize their health and well-being:

1. **Improved Respiratory Health**: By promoting mucus clearance and supporting lung function, Dr. Barbara's approach can alleviate congestion, reduce coughing, and enhance respiratory comfort. Herbal remedies such as expectorants, demulcents, and lung tonics help to soothe irritated mucous membranes and promote healthy respiratory function.

2. **Enhanced Digestive Function**: A mucus cleanse can support digestive health by reducing congestion in the gastrointestinal tract and promoting optimal nutrient absorption. Herbal remedies such as bitter tonics, digestive aids, and carminatives help to stimulate digestion, alleviate bloating, and improve bowel regularity, leading to greater comfort and vitality.

3. **Immune Support**: Many herbs possess immune-modulating properties that can strengthen the body's natural defenses and promote resilience against infections. By incorporating immune-supportive herbs into her protocols, Dr. Barbara helps individuals bolster their immune function and reduce the risk of illness, especially during periods of heightened susceptibility.

4. **Overall Vitality and Well-being**: By addressing underlying imbalances and supporting the body's natural healing mechanisms, Dr. Barbara's approach promotes a sense of vitality, resilience, and well-being. Individuals who adopt her holistic protocols often report increased energy levels, improved mood, and a greater capacity to cope with stress, leading to a higher quality of life.

In conclusion, Dr. Barbara's approach to herbal healing and mucus cleanse offers a holistic framework for promoting health and vitality naturally. By integrating traditional wisdom, scientific knowledge, and personalized care, she empowers individuals to take charge of their health and embark on a journey of healing and transformation. Whether seeking relief from respiratory congestion, digestive discomfort, or immune challenges, individuals can benefit from Dr. Barbara's expertise and guidance in achieving optimal wellness through herbal healing and mucus cleanse.

CHAPTER TWO

Understanding the Role of Mucus in the Body's Health

Mucus is often viewed with disdain, associated with nasal congestion, coughing fits, and unpleasant bodily secretions. However, this seemingly humble substance plays a crucial role in maintaining the body's health and protecting against infections and environmental threats. In this comprehensive exploration, we'll delve into the multifaceted functions of mucus, its composition, production, and its significance in supporting respiratory, gastrointestinal, and reproductive health.

The Composition of Mucus

Mucus is a gel-like substance produced by specialized cells known as goblet cells, which are found in the epithelial lining of various organs, including the respiratory tract, gastrointestinal tract, and reproductive organs. It consists primarily of water, mucins (glycoproteins), electrolytes, enzymes, and immunoglobulins (antibodies). The exact composition of mucus varies depending on its location in the body and its specific physiological function.

Mucins are the key structural components of mucus, forming a network of glycoprotein chains that give mucus its gel-like consistency and adhesive properties. These mucin molecules can trap pathogens, allergens, and particulate matter, preventing them from reaching vulnerable tissues and initiating infection or inflammation. Additionally, mucus contains enzymes such as lysozyme, lactoferrin, and immunoglobulins, which have antimicrobial properties and help to neutralize pathogens.

The Protective Functions of Mucus

Mucus serves as a critical barrier against external threats, providing a first line of defense against infections, toxins, and mechanical damage. Its viscoelastic properties enable it to trap and immobilize pathogens, preventing them from adhering to epithelial surfaces and penetrating underlying tissues. By forming a physical barrier, mucus helps to shield vulnerable tissues from irritants, pollutants, and abrasive particles, reducing the risk of inflammation and tissue damage.

In the respiratory tract, mucus acts as a filter, humidifier, and lubricant, trapping airborne particles, moisturizing the airway lining, and facilitating the clearance of mucus from the lungs. In the gastrointestinal tract, mucus protects the delicate mucous membranes from digestive enzymes, acid, and abrasive food particles, while also facilitating the movement of food through the digestive system. In the reproductive tract, cervical mucus plays a vital role in fertility and conception by providing a hospitable environment for sperm transport and protecting against microbial invasion.

Regulation of Mucus Production

The production and secretion of mucus are tightly regulated by various factors, including hormonal signals, neural inputs, immune mediators, and environmental stimuli. In response to microbial infections, allergens, or inflammatory stimuli, the body may increase mucus production as part of the immune response to clear pathogens and promote tissue repair. Conversely, certain conditions such as dehydration, smoking, or environmental pollutants can impair mucus production and clearance, leading to mucosal dryness and dysfunction.

Dysregulation of Mucus in Disease

Disorders of mucus production or clearance can have profound implications for health, predisposing individuals to respiratory infections, gastrointestinal disorders, and reproductive problems. Conditions such as cystic fibrosis, chronic obstructive pulmonary disease (COPD), asthma, and inflammatory bowel disease (IBD) are characterized by abnormalities in mucus secretion, viscosity, or clearance mechanisms, leading to mucus buildup, inflammation, and tissue damage.

In cystic fibrosis, for example, mutations in the cystic fibrosis transmembrane conductance regulator (CFTR) gene impair chloride ion transport across epithelial cells, resulting in thick, sticky mucus that obstructs the airways and predisposes individuals to recurrent respiratory infections. Similarly, in IBD, chronic inflammation of the intestinal mucosa disrupts the integrity of the mucus layer, allowing luminal bacteria to penetrate the epithelial barrier and trigger inflammatory responses.

Clinical Implications and Therapeutic Interventions

Understanding the role of mucus in health and disease has important clinical implications for the diagnosis, treatment, and prevention of various disorders. Therapeutic interventions aimed at modulating mucus production, composition, or clearance mechanisms may offer promising avenues for managing respiratory conditions, gastrointestinal diseases, and reproductive disorders.

For example, mucolytic agents such as acetylcysteine and guaifenesin can help to thin and liquefy thickened mucus, making it easier to expectorate and clear from the airways. Mucokinetic agents such as hypertonic saline and mannitol can enhance mucociliary clearance by promoting the hydration and mobilization of mucus in the respiratory tract. In addition, dietary modifications, hydration, and lifestyle changes may play a crucial role in supporting healthy mucus production and function, reducing the risk of mucosal dysfunction and associated complications.

In conclusion, mucus plays a multifaceted role in maintaining the body's health and protecting against infections and environmental threats. Its composition, production, and clearance mechanisms are tightly regulated by various factors, and dysregulation of mucus homeostasis can contribute to the pathogenesis of numerous diseases. By understanding the physiological functions of mucus and its clinical implications, healthcare providers can develop targeted interventions to optimize mucus health and promote overall well-being.

CHAPTER THREE

The Connection Between Diet, Lifestyle, and Mucus Production

Mucus production is a fundamental physiological process that plays a crucial role in protecting the body's mucous membranes and maintaining respiratory, gastrointestinal, and reproductive health. While mucus production is primarily regulated by genetic and physiological factors, emerging evidence suggests that diet and lifestyle factors can also influence mucus secretion, composition, and clearance mechanisms. In this comprehensive exploration, we'll delve into the intricate connection between diet, lifestyle, and mucus production, examining how dietary choices, hydration status, environmental exposures, and other lifestyle factors can impact mucus health and function.

Dietary Influence on Mucus Production

Dietary factors play a significant role in modulating mucus production and composition, with certain foods and nutrients exerting pro-inflammatory or anti-inflammatory effects on mucous membranes. For example, a diet high in processed foods, refined sugars, and saturated fats has been associated with increased inflammation and mucus production in the respiratory and gastrointestinal tracts. Conversely, a diet rich in fruits, vegetables, whole grains, and omega-3 fatty acids has been shown to have anti-inflammatory effects and may help to reduce excessive mucus production.

Specific nutrients, such as vitamin C, vitamin E, zinc, and selenium, play important roles in supporting mucosal health and immune function. These micronutrients act as antioxidants, scavenging free radicals and protecting mucous membranes from oxidative damage. Adequate hydration is also essential for maintaining optimal mucus viscosity and clearance, as dehydration can lead to thickened, inspissated mucus that impairs mucociliary clearance and predisposes individuals to respiratory and gastrointestinal problems.

Impact of Lifestyle Factors on Mucus Production

In addition to dietary choices, various lifestyle factors can influence mucus production, viscosity, and clearance mechanisms. Chronic stress, for example, has been shown to dysregulate the hypothalamic-pituitary-adrenal (HPA) axis and increase circulating levels of cortisol, which can suppress immune function and promote inflammation in mucous membranes. Sleep deprivation, sedentary behavior, and exposure to environmental pollutants such as tobacco smoke, air pollution, and allergens can also exacerbate mucosal inflammation and mucus hypersecretion.

Conversely, regular physical activity, adequate sleep, stress management techniques, and avoidance of environmental toxins can help to support mucosal health and reduce the risk of excessive mucus production. Mind-body practices such as yoga, meditation, and deep breathing exercises may also have beneficial effects on mucociliary clearance and respiratory function by promoting relaxation, reducing stress, and enhancing immune function.

Role of Hydration in Mucus Health

Proper hydration is essential for maintaining optimal mucus viscosity and facilitating mucociliary clearance in the respiratory and gastrointestinal tracts. Water acts as a lubricant, helping to keep mucus thin and slippery, which promotes effective clearance of mucus from the body. Dehydration, on the other hand, can lead to thickened, sticky mucus that is difficult to clear, increasing the risk of respiratory infections, gastrointestinal disorders, and other mucosal problems.

In addition to water, certain beverages such as herbal teas, broths, and warm fluids can help to hydrate the body and support mucus health. However, it's important to avoid excessive consumption of sugary beverages, caffeine, and alcohol, as these substances can dehydrate the body and exacerbate mucosal dryness and irritation.

Practical Strategies for Supporting Mucus Health

Based on the interconnectedness of diet, lifestyle, and mucus production, several practical strategies can be implemented to support optimal mucus health and function:

1. **Adopt a Balanced Diet**: Focus on consuming a diet rich in fruits, vegetables, whole grains, and healthy fats to provide essential nutrients and antioxidants that support mucosal health and reduce inflammation.

2. **Stay Hydrated**: Drink an adequate amount of water throughout the day to keep mucus thin and lubricated, facilitating effective clearance from the body.

3. **Manage Stress**: Incorporate stress management techniques such as mindfulness meditation, deep breathing exercises, and progressive muscle relaxation to reduce stress levels and support immune function.

4. **Get Regular Exercise**: Engage in regular physical activity to promote circulation, enhance immune function, and support mucosal health.

5. **Avoid Environmental Toxins**: Minimize exposure to environmental pollutants, allergens, and irritants such as tobacco smoke, air pollution, and chemical fumes that can

exacerbate mucosal inflammation and mucus hypersecretion.

By adopting these lifestyle practices and dietary habits, individuals can promote optimal mucus health and reduce the risk of respiratory, gastrointestinal, and reproductive disorders associated with mucus dysfunction. Taking a holistic approach that addresses the interconnectedness of diet, lifestyle, and mucus production can help to optimize overall health and well-being.

CHAPTER FOUR

Dr. Barbara's Principles of Herbal Medicine and Mucus Reduction

Dr. Barbara's approach to herbal medicine and mucus reduction is rooted in the principles of holistic health, traditional herbalism, and evidence-based practice. With a deep understanding of the body's innate healing mechanisms and the therapeutic properties of medicinal plants, Dr. Barbara employs a comprehensive approach to address mucus-related concerns and promote overall wellness. In this detailed exploration, we'll delve into the fundamental principles that guide Dr. Barbara's practice of herbal medicine and mucus reduction, including the selection of appropriate herbs, therapeutic strategies, and lifestyle interventions.

Holistic Approach to Health

Central to Dr. Barbara's principles is the recognition that health is a multifaceted interplay of physical, emotional, and spiritual well-being. Rather than simply treating symptoms, Dr. Barbara takes a holistic approach that considers the underlying imbalances and root causes of illness. She views the body as a dynamic ecosystem, with each organ system interconnected and influenced by various factors, including diet, lifestyle, environment, and mindset.

In addressing mucus-related concerns, Dr. Barbara looks beyond symptomatic relief to identify and address the underlying factors contributing to excessive mucus production or impaired clearance. This holistic perspective allows her to develop personalized treatment plans that support the body's natural healing processes and promote long-term wellness.

Traditional Herbalism and Plant Medicine

Dr. Barbara draws upon the rich tradition of herbalism and plant medicine, recognizing the therapeutic potential of medicinal plants in promoting health and alleviating symptoms. Throughout history, cultures worldwide have relied on herbs for their healing properties, passing down knowledge of herbal remedies through generations. Dr. Barbara combines traditional wisdom with modern scientific research to identify herbs that are effective in reducing mucus production, thinning mucus secretions, and supporting respiratory and gastrointestinal health.

Herbal remedies may be administered in various forms, including teas, tinctures, capsules, and topical preparations, depending on the individual's preferences and therapeutic goals. Dr. Barbara selects herbs based on their specific actions and indications, taking into account factors such as the herb's botanical properties, chemical constituents, pharmacological effects, and safety profile.

Mucus Reduction Strategies

In addressing mucus-related concerns, Dr. Barbara employs a multifaceted approach that targets both the symptoms and underlying imbalances contributing to mucus accumulation. Her mucus reduction strategies may include:

1. **Mucolytic Herbs**: Dr. Barbara selects herbs with mucolytic properties that help to thin and liquefy thickened mucus, making it easier to expel from the body. Common mucolytic herbs include mullein leaf, elecampane root, thyme, and licorice root.

2. **Expectorant Herbs**: Expectorant herbs promote the expulsion of mucus from the respiratory tract by stimulating coughing and increasing bronchial secretions. Herbs such as hyssop, coltsfoot, wild cherry bark, and eucalyptus are often used to support respiratory health and relieve congestion.

3. **Demulcent Herbs**: Demulcent herbs soothe and protect irritated mucous membranes, reducing inflammation and promoting healing. These herbs form a protective layer over mucosal tissues, providing relief from dryness, irritation, and inflammation. Common demulcent herbs include marshmallow root, slippery elm bark, licorice root, and plantain leaf.

4. **Anti-inflammatory Herbs**: Inflammation often accompanies excessive mucus production and can exacerbate symptoms

of respiratory and gastrointestinal disorders. Dr. Barbara selects anti-inflammatory herbs such as turmeric, ginger, boswellia, and chamomile to reduce inflammation and soothe irritated tissues.

5. **Immune-supportive Herbs**: Supporting immune function is essential for resolving mucus-related concerns and preventing recurrent infections. Dr. Barbara incorporates immune-supportive herbs such as echinacea, astragalus, elderberry, and medicinal mushrooms to strengthen the body's natural defenses and promote resilience against infections.

Lifestyle Recommendations

In addition to herbal remedies, Dr. Barbara emphasizes the importance of lifestyle interventions in mucus reduction and overall health promotion. Lifestyle recommendations may include:

- **Dietary Modifications**: Adopting a balanced diet rich in fruits, vegetables, whole grains, and lean proteins can support mucus reduction and promote immune function. Avoiding inflammatory foods such as processed foods, refined sugars, and trans fats can help to reduce mucus production and inflammation.

- **Hydration**: Adequate hydration is crucial for maintaining optimal mucus viscosity and promoting mucociliary clearance. Dr. Barbara recommends drinking plenty of water throughout the day and consuming hydrating beverages such as herbal teas, broths, and fresh juices.

- **Stress Management**: Chronic stress can dysregulate the immune system and exacerbate mucus-related symptoms. Dr. Barbara encourages stress management techniques such as meditation, deep breathing exercises, yoga, and mindfulness practices to promote relaxation and reduce stress.

- **Physical Activity**: Regular exercise supports immune function, enhances circulation, and promotes respiratory health. Dr. Barbara recommends incorporating physical activity into daily routines, such as walking, jogging, swimming, or yoga, to support mucus reduction and overall well-being.

By integrating herbal medicine, mucus reduction strategies, and lifestyle interventions, Dr. Barbara provides a holistic approach to health that addresses the root causes of mucus-related concerns and supports the body's natural healing processes. Her principles of herbal medicine and mucus reduction empower individuals to take charge of their health and achieve optimal wellness through natural, holistic means.

CHAPTER FIVE

Preparing Your Body and Mind for the Herbal Mucus Cleanse

Embarking on a herbal mucus cleanse involves more than simply consuming herbal remedies; it requires a holistic approach that encompasses both physical and mental preparation. By preparing your body and mind adequately, you can optimize the effectiveness of the cleanse and promote overall well-being. In this comprehensive guide, we'll explore the essential steps and considerations for preparing your body and mind for a herbal mucus cleanse.

Understanding the Purpose of the Cleanse

Before beginning a herbal mucus cleanse, it's essential to understand its purpose and potential benefits. A mucus cleanse aims to support the body's natural detoxification processes, facilitate the elimination of excess mucus, and promote respiratory, gastrointestinal, and overall health. By clearing accumulated mucus from the body, individuals may experience improved breathing, digestion, energy levels, and vitality. Understanding the goals of the cleanse can provide motivation and clarity as you prepare for the process.

Consulting with a Healthcare Professional

Before starting any cleanse or detoxification program, it's crucial to consult with a qualified healthcare professional, especially if you have underlying health conditions or are taking medications. A healthcare provider can assess your individual health status, provide personalized recommendations, and ensure that the cleanse is safe and appropriate for you. They can also offer guidance on potential contraindications, dosage adjustments, and monitoring during the cleanse process.

Setting Realistic Goals and Expectations

Setting realistic goals and expectations is key to a successful cleanse experience. While a herbal mucus cleanse can offer numerous benefits, it's essential to understand that it is not a quick fix or a cure-all solution. Results may vary depending on individual factors such as health status, lifestyle habits, and adherence to the cleanse protocol. By setting achievable goals and maintaining a positive mindset, you can approach the cleanse with realistic expectations and enhance your overall experience.

Preparing Your Diet

Dietary preparation is a crucial aspect of preparing your body for a herbal mucus cleanse. Begin by gradually transitioning to a clean, whole foods-based diet rich in fruits, vegetables, whole grains, lean proteins, and healthy fats. Minimize or eliminate processed foods, refined sugars, artificial additives, and inflammatory ingredients that may exacerbate mucus production and impair detoxification processes.

Incorporate hydrating foods such as cucumbers, celery, watermelon, and citrus fruits to support mucus clearance and maintain optimal hydration levels. Consider incorporating herbal teas, broths, and fresh juices into your daily routine to nourish your body and prepare it for the cleanse process. Additionally, consider reducing or eliminating caffeine, alcohol, and stimulants to support detoxification and promote relaxation.

Hydration and Hygiene Practices

Proper hydration and hygiene practices are essential for supporting the body's natural detoxification processes and promoting overall health. Increase your water intake in the days leading up to the cleanse to ensure adequate hydration and support mucus clearance. Aim to drink at least eight glasses of water per day, and consider incorporating hydrating beverages such as herbal teas, coconut water, and electrolyte-rich drinks.

Practice good hygiene habits, including regular handwashing, oral hygiene, and nasal irrigation, to reduce the risk of infections and support respiratory health. Consider using a saline nasal spray or neti pot to flush out excess mucus and allergens from the nasal passages, promoting clearer breathing and reducing congestion.

Mindful Practices and Stress Management

Preparing your mind for a herbal mucus cleanse involves cultivating a mindset of mindfulness, self-awareness, and relaxation. Engage in mindful practices such as meditation, deep breathing exercises, yoga, or tai chi to reduce stress, promote mental clarity, and enhance your overall well-being. Set aside time each day for self-care activities that nourish your mind, body, and spirit, such as taking nature walks, journaling, or listening to soothing music.

Address any underlying stressors or emotional imbalances that may impact your health and well-being. Consider seeking support from a therapist, counselor, or support group to explore coping strategies, process emotions, and cultivate resilience during the cleanse process. By prioritizing self-care and stress management, you can create a supportive environment for your body to undergo the cleanse and promote optimal outcomes.

Conclusion

Preparing your body and mind for a herbal mucus cleanse involves a comprehensive approach that addresses dietary, lifestyle, and psychological factors. By understanding the purpose of the cleanse, consulting with a healthcare professional, setting realistic goals, and adopting supportive practices, you can optimize the effectiveness of the cleanse and promote overall health and well-being. With careful preparation and mindful attention, you can embark on the cleanse journey with confidence, clarity, and a sense of empowerment to support your body's natural healing processes.

CHAPTER SIX

Selecting the Right Herbs for Mucus Reduction and Detoxification

Choosing the appropriate herbs for mucus reduction and detoxification is a crucial step in creating an effective herbal cleanse protocol. By selecting herbs with specific therapeutic properties and actions, you can support the body's natural detoxification processes, promote mucus clearance, and enhance overall well-being. In this comprehensive guide, we'll explore key factors to consider when selecting herbs for mucus reduction and detoxification, as well as a selection of herbs known for their beneficial effects on respiratory, gastrointestinal, and immune health.

Understanding Herbal Actions and Properties

Before choosing herbs for mucus reduction and detoxification, it's important to understand their various actions and properties. Herbs can have diverse therapeutic effects on the body, including mucolytic, expectorant, demulcent, anti-inflammatory, immune-supportive, and detoxifying properties. By selecting herbs with complementary actions, you can create a synergistic blend that addresses multiple aspects of mucus-related concerns and supports overall health.

- **Mucolytic Herbs**: Mucolytic herbs help to thin and liquefy thickened mucus, making it easier to expel from the body. These herbs often contain enzymes or compounds that break down the structural components of mucus, such as glycoproteins. Examples of mucolytic herbs include mullein leaf, elecampane root, thyme, and fenugreek seed.

- **Expectorant Herbs**: Expectorant herbs promote the expulsion of mucus from the respiratory tract by stimulating coughing and increasing bronchial secretions. These herbs help to clear congested airways and facilitate mucus clearance. Common expectorant herbs include hyssop, coltsfoot, wild cherry bark, and eucalyptus.

- **Demulcent Herbs**: Demulcent herbs soothe and protect irritated mucous membranes, reducing inflammation and promoting healing. These herbs form a protective layer over mucosal tissues, providing relief from dryness, irritation, and inflammation. Examples of demulcent herbs include marshmallow root, slippery elm bark, licorice root, and plantain leaf.

- **Anti-inflammatory Herbs**: Anti-inflammatory herbs help to reduce inflammation in the respiratory and gastrointestinal tracts, alleviating symptoms such as congestion, irritation, and discomfort. These herbs may inhibit inflammatory pathways and modulate immune responses. Common anti-inflammatory herbs include turmeric, ginger, boswellia, and chamomile.

- **Immune-supportive Herbs**: Supporting immune function is essential for detoxification and overall health. Immune-supportive herbs help to strengthen the body's natural defenses and promote resilience against infections. Examples of immune-supportive herbs include echinacea, astragalus, elderberry, and medicinal mushrooms.

Considerations for Herb Selection

When selecting herbs for mucus reduction and detoxification, it's important to consider several factors:

1. **Individual Health Status**: Take into account your individual health status, including any underlying health conditions, medications, allergies, or sensitivities. Consult with a qualified healthcare professional to ensure that the selected herbs are safe and appropriate for your specific needs.

2. **Therapeutic Goals**: Identify your therapeutic goals and desired outcomes for the herbal cleanse. Are you primarily seeking to reduce respiratory congestion, support gastrointestinal health, boost immune function, or promote overall detoxification? Tailor your herb selection to align with your specific goals and concerns.

3. **Herb Interactions**: Be mindful of potential interactions between herbs and medications or other supplements you may be taking. Some herbs may interact with certain medications, altering their effectiveness or causing adverse effects. Research potential herb-drug interactions or consult with a healthcare provider for personalized guidance.

4. **Quality and Purity**: Choose high-quality, organic herbs from reputable sources to ensure purity, potency, and safety. Look for herbs that have been tested for contaminants and standardized for active constituents. Consider purchasing herbs in whole form and preparing your own herbal preparations for maximum freshness and efficacy.

Sample Herbal Selections

Here are some examples of herbs commonly used for mucus reduction and detoxification:

1. **Mullein Leaf (Verbascum thapsus)**: A mucolytic and expectorant herb that helps to loosen and expel thickened mucus from the respiratory tract.

2. **Marshmallow Root (Althaea officinalis)**: A demulcent herb that soothes and protects irritated mucous membranes in the respiratory and gastrointestinal tracts.

3. **Elderberry (Sambucus nigra)**: An immune-supportive herb rich in antioxidants and flavonoids that help to strengthen the immune system and reduce inflammation.

4. **Turmeric (Curcuma longa)**: An anti-inflammatory herb with potent antioxidant properties that supports detoxification and reduces inflammation in the body.

5. **Ginger (Zingiber officinale)**: An expectorant and anti-inflammatory herb that helps to clear congestion, soothe sore throats, and support digestive health.

6. **Echinacea (Echinacea spp.)**: An immune-supportive herb that enhances immune function and promotes resistance to infections, particularly in the respiratory tract.

Conclusion

Selecting the right herbs for mucus reduction and detoxification involves considering their therapeutic actions, individual health status, therapeutic goals, potential herb interactions, and quality standards. By choosing herbs with complementary properties and aligning them with your specific needs and preferences, you can create a customized herbal cleanse protocol that supports optimal health and well-being. Always consult with a qualified healthcare professional before starting any herbal cleanse or detoxification program, especially if you have underlying health conditions or are taking medications. With careful selection and mindful attention, herbal medicine can be a powerful tool for promoting mucus reduction, detoxification, and overall vitality.

CHAPTER SEVEN

Herbal Remedies and Formulations for Clearing Excess Mucus

Excess mucus production can lead to respiratory congestion, throat irritation, and digestive discomfort, among other symptoms. Herbal remedies offer a natural and effective approach to clearing excess mucus from the body, supporting respiratory and gastrointestinal health, and promoting overall well-being. In this comprehensive guide, we'll explore various herbal remedies and formulations known for their mucolytic, expectorant, demulcent, and anti-inflammatory properties, as well as sample formulations for clearing excess mucus.

Mucolytic Herbs

Mucolytic herbs help to thin and liquefy thickened mucus, making it easier to expel from the body. These herbs contain enzymes or compounds that break down the structural components of mucus, such as glycoproteins.

1. **Mullein Leaf (Verbascum thapsus)**: Mullein is a mucolytic herb with expectorant properties that help to loosen and expel thickened mucus from the respiratory tract. It can be used as a tea, tincture, or steam inhalation.

2. **Elecampane Root (Inula helenium)**: Elecampane is a powerful mucolytic herb that helps to clear congestion in the

lungs and promote expectoration of mucus. It can be taken as a tea, tincture, or syrup.

3. **Thyme (Thymus vulgaris)**: Thyme is rich in volatile oils with expectorant and antimicrobial properties that help to relieve respiratory congestion and promote mucus clearance. It can be used in teas, tinctures, or as a steam inhalation.

Expectorant Herbs

Expectorant herbs promote the expulsion of mucus from the respiratory tract by stimulating coughing and increasing bronchial secretions.

1. **Hyssop (Hyssopus officinalis)**: Hyssop is an expectorant herb that helps to clear congestion in the lungs and promote productive coughing to expel mucus. It can be used as a tea, tincture, or syrup.

2. **Coltsfoot (Tussilago farfara)**: Coltsfoot is a traditional remedy for respiratory conditions characterized by excessive mucus production. It helps to soothe irritated mucous membranes and promote expectoration. It can be taken as a tea, tincture, or syrup.

3. **Wild Cherry Bark (Prunus serotina)**: Wild cherry bark is a gentle expectorant that helps to loosen and expel mucus from the respiratory tract. It can be used as a tea, tincture, or syrup.

Demulcent Herbs

Demulcent herbs soothe and protect irritated mucous membranes, reducing inflammation and promoting healing.

1. **Marshmallow Root (Althaea officinalis)**: Marshmallow root is a demulcent herb that forms a protective coating over mucous membranes, providing relief from irritation and inflammation. It can be taken as a tea, tincture, or syrup.

2. **Slippery Elm Bark (Ulmus rubra)**: Slippery elm bark is rich in mucilage, a gel-like substance that soothes and protects the lining of the respiratory and gastrointestinal tracts. It can be used as a tea, powder, or lozenge.

3. **Licorice Root (Glycyrrhiza glabra)**: Licorice root is a demulcent and expectorant herb that helps to soothe sore throats, reduce coughing, and clear congestion in the lungs. It can be taken as a tea, tincture, or syrup.

Anti-inflammatory Herbs

Anti-inflammatory herbs help to reduce inflammation in the respiratory and gastrointestinal tracts, alleviating symptoms such as congestion, irritation, and discomfort.

1. **Turmeric (Curcuma longa)**: Turmeric is a potent anti-inflammatory herb that helps to reduce inflammation and irritation in the respiratory and gastrointestinal tracts. It can be taken as a tea, capsule, or added to food as a spice.

2. **Ginger (Zingiber officinale)**: Ginger is a warming herb with anti-inflammatory properties that help to soothe respiratory and digestive discomfort. It can be used in teas, tinctures, or added to food as a spice.

3. **Chamomile (Matricaria chamomilla)**: Chamomile is a gentle anti-inflammatory herb that helps to calm and soothe irritated mucous membranes in the respiratory and gastrointestinal tracts. It can be taken as a tea or tincture.

Sample Herbal Formulations

Here are some sample herbal formulations for clearing excess mucus:

1. **Respiratory Relief Tea**: Mix equal parts of mullein leaf, elecampane root, and thyme. Steep 1 tablespoon of the herb blend in hot water for 10-15 minutes. Drink 2-3 cups daily to help clear respiratory congestion and promote mucus clearance.

2. **Mucus-Busting Syrup**: Combine equal parts of licorice root, marshmallow root, and wild cherry bark. Simmer the herbs in water for 30-40 minutes to make a strong decoction. Strain the liquid and add honey to taste. Take 1-2 teaspoons of the syrup as needed to relieve coughing and promote expectoration.

3. **Digestive Comfort Tincture**: Mix equal parts of ginger root, chamomile flowers, and fennel seeds. Fill a jar with the herb blend and cover with vodka or another high-proof alcohol. Let the mixture steep for 4-6 weeks, shaking daily. Strain the liquid and take 1-2 dropperfuls before meals to support digestion and reduce gastrointestinal discomfort.

Conclusion

Herbal remedies offer a natural and effective approach to clearing excess mucus from the body and promoting respiratory, gastrointestinal, and overall health. By selecting herbs with mucolytic, expectorant, demulcent, and anti-inflammatory properties, you can create personalized formulations to address your specific needs and preferences. Consult with a qualified herbalist or healthcare professional for personalized guidance and recommendations tailored to your individual health status and goals. With the right herbal remedies and formulations, you can support your body's natural detoxification processes and enjoy improved well-being.

CHAPTER EIGHT

Incorporating Herbal Teas and Supplements for Enhanced Cleanse Results

Herbal teas and supplements can be valuable additions to a mucus cleanse regimen, offering targeted support for detoxification, mucus reduction, and overall well-being. By incorporating specific herbs and supplements into your cleanse protocol, you can enhance the effectiveness of the cleanse and promote optimal results. In this guide, we'll explore the benefits of herbal teas and supplements for mucus reduction, detoxification, and respiratory health, as well as practical tips for incorporating them into your cleanse routine.

Benefits of Herbal Teas and Supplements

Herbal teas and supplements offer a convenient and enjoyable way to consume beneficial herbs and nutrients that support mucus reduction, detoxification, and respiratory health. They can provide concentrated doses of key compounds that help to thin mucus, clear congestion, soothe irritated mucous membranes, and promote overall wellness. Additionally, herbal teas and supplements are easy to incorporate into daily routines and can be customized to address specific health concerns and preferences.

Mucus-Reducing Herbal Teas

Certain herbal teas are particularly well-suited for reducing excess mucus and supporting respiratory health. These teas often contain mucolytic, expectorant, and anti-inflammatory herbs that help to thin mucus, clear congestion, and soothe respiratory discomfort. Here are some examples of mucus-reducing herbal teas:

1. **Peppermint Tea**: Peppermint contains menthol, which has a cooling effect on the respiratory tract and helps to alleviate congestion and promote easier breathing.

2. **Ginger Tea**: Ginger is a warming herb with anti-inflammatory properties that help to reduce inflammation in the respiratory tract and promote mucus clearance.

3. **Eucalyptus Tea**: Eucalyptus contains cineole, a compound with expectorant properties that help to loosen mucus and clear congestion in the lungs.

4. **Licorice Root Tea**: Licorice root is a demulcent herb that soothes irritated mucous membranes and helps to reduce inflammation in the respiratory tract.

Detoxifying Herbal Supplements

In addition to herbal teas, certain herbal supplements can support detoxification and enhance the body's natural cleansing processes. These supplements often contain herbs and nutrients that promote liver function, support digestion, and eliminate toxins from the body. Here are some examples of detoxifying herbal supplements:

1. **Milk Thistle**: Milk thistle is a liver-supportive herb that helps to protect and regenerate liver cells, promote detoxification, and eliminate toxins from the body.

2. **Dandelion Root**: Dandelion root is a diuretic herb that supports kidney function and helps to eliminate waste products and toxins from the body through urine.

3. **Burdock Root**: Burdock root is a blood-cleansing herb that helps to eliminate toxins from the bloodstream, support lymphatic drainage, and promote overall detoxification.

4. **Nettle Leaf**: Nettle leaf is a nutritive herb rich in vitamins, minerals, and antioxidants that support kidney function, promote detoxification, and reduce inflammation in the body.

DR. BARBARA RECIPES FOR MUCUS CLEANSE

1. Lemon Ginger Tea:

- **Definition:** Lemon ginger tea is a soothing beverage known for its ability to clear congestion and promote healthy digestion.

- **Ingredients:** Fresh ginger, lemon juice, honey, water.

- **How to Prepare:** Grate ginger into boiling water, add lemon juice and honey, simmer for a few minutes.

- **How to Use:** Drink 1-2 cups daily.

- **Dosage:** 1-2 cups per day.

- **Side Effect:** May cause heartburn or upset stomach in some individuals.

- **Precaution:** Avoid if allergic to any ingredients.

2. Turmeric Milk:

- **Definition:** Turmeric milk is an ancient remedy for respiratory ailments and inflammation.

- **Ingredients:** Turmeric powder, milk, honey.

- **How to Prepare:** Heat milk, add turmeric and honey, simmer for a few minutes.

- **How to Use:** Drink before bedtime.

- o **Dosage:** 1 cup per day.

- o **Side Effect:** Rarely, may cause gastrointestinal issues or allergic reactions.

- o **Precaution:** Avoid excessive consumption.

3. Apple Cider Vinegar Drink:

- o **Definition:** Apple cider vinegar helps break down mucus and promotes detoxification.

- o **Ingredients:** Apple cider vinegar, water, honey.

- o **How to Prepare:** Mix apple cider vinegar and honey in warm water.

- o **How to Use:** Drink on an empty stomach.

- o **Dosage:** 1-2 tablespoons diluted in water daily.

- o **Side Effect:** May erode tooth enamel or cause throat irritation if not diluted properly.

- o **Precaution:** Rinse mouth after consumption.

4. Eucalyptus Steam Inhalation:

- o **Definition:** Eucalyptus steam inhalation helps clear nasal passages and relieve congestion.

- o **Ingredients:** Eucalyptus essential oil, boiling water.

- o **How to Prepare:** Add a few drops of eucalyptus oil to boiling water, inhale steam with a towel over your head.

- o **How to Use:** Inhale steam for 5-10 minutes.

- o **Dosage:** Once daily.

- o **Side Effect:** May cause skin irritation if oil comes into direct contact.

- o **Precaution:** Keep eyes closed during inhalation.

5. Nettle Leaf Tea:

- o **Definition:** Nettle leaf tea is a natural antihistamine that reduces mucus production.

- o **Ingredients:** Dried nettle leaves, boiling water.

- o **How to Prepare:** Steep nettle leaves in boiling water for 5-10 minutes.

- o **How to Use:** Drink 1-2 cups daily.

- o **Dosage:** 1-2 cups per day.

- o **Side Effect:** May cause mild stomach upset or allergic reactions in sensitive individuals.

- o **Precaution:** Avoid if pregnant or allergic to plants in the Urticaceae family.

6. **Peppermint Tea:**

   - **Definition:** Peppermint tea acts as a decongestant and soothes irritated airways.

   - **Ingredients:** Peppermint leaves, boiling water.

   - **How to Prepare:** Steep peppermint leaves in boiling water for 5-10 minutes.

   - **How to Use:** Drink 1-2 cups daily.

   - **Dosage:** 1-2 cups per day.

   - **Side Effect:** May cause heartburn or acid reflux in some individuals.

   - **Precaution:** Avoid if suffering from gastroesophageal reflux disease (GERD).

7. **Garlic Soup:**

   - **Definition:** Garlic soup boosts immunity and has antimicrobial properties.

   - **Ingredients:** Garlic cloves, vegetable broth, onions, olive oil.

   - **How to Prepare:** Sauté garlic and onions in olive oil, add vegetable broth, simmer until garlic is soft.

   - **How to Use:** Consume as a soup.

- **Dosage:** 1 bowl per day.
- **Side Effect:** May cause bad breath or digestive discomfort.
- **Precaution:** Avoid if allergic to garlic or onions.

8. Cayenne Pepper Lemonade:

- **Definition:** Cayenne pepper lemonade stimulates circulation and loosens mucus.
- **Ingredients:** Cayenne pepper, lemon juice, maple syrup, water.
- **How to Prepare:** Mix lemon juice, maple syrup, and a pinch of cayenne pepper in water.
- **How to Use:** Drink throughout the day.
- **Dosage:** As desired.
- **Side Effect:** May cause stomach irritation or increased heartburn.
- **Precaution:** Start with a small amount of cayenne pepper.

9. Green Smoothie:

- **Definition:** Green smoothies are packed with nutrients and antioxidants that support respiratory health.

- o **Ingredients:** Spinach, kale, banana, pineapple, coconut water.

- o **How to Prepare:** Blend all ingredients until smooth.

- o **How to Use:** Drink as a meal replacement or snack.

- o **Dosage:** 1-2 servings per day.

- o **Side Effect:** None when consumed in moderation.

- o **Precaution:** Avoid if allergic to any ingredients.

10. **Fenugreek Tea:**

- o **Definition:** Fenugreek tea thins mucus and relieves respiratory congestion.

- o **Ingredients:** Fenugreek seeds, boiling water, honey.

- o **How to Prepare:** Steep fenugreek seeds in boiling water for 10-15 minutes, add honey if desired.

- o **How to Use:** Drink 1-2 cups daily.

- o **Dosage:** 1-2 cups per day.

- o **Side Effect:** May cause nausea or diarrhea in large amounts.

- o **Precaution:** Avoid if pregnant or allergic to fenugreek.

11. **Licorice Root Tea:**

- **Definition:** Licorice root tea soothes throat irritation and reduces mucus production.

- **Ingredients:** Dried licorice root, boiling water, honey (optional).

- **How to Prepare:** Steep licorice root in boiling water for 5-10 minutes, add honey if desired.

- **How to Use:** Drink 1-2 cups daily.

- **Dosage:** 1-2 cups per day.

- **Side Effect:** Prolonged use may lead to high blood pressure or potassium depletion.

- **Precaution:** Avoid if pregnant, diabetic, or have hypertension.

12. **Honey Lemon Water:**

- **Definition:** Honey lemon water hydrates the body and soothes sore throats.

- **Ingredients:** Lemon juice, honey, warm water.

- **How to Prepare:** Mix lemon juice and honey in warm water.

- **How to Use:** Drink in the morning on an empty stomach.

- **Dosage:** 1 glass per day.

- **Side Effect:** Rarely, may cause allergic reactions in sensitive individuals.

- **Precaution:** Use raw honey for maximum benefits.

13. **Onion Syrup:**

- **Definition:** Onion syrup has expectorant properties and helps eliminate mucus from the respiratory tract.

- **Ingredients:** Onion, honey.

- **How to Prepare:** Slice onion and layer it with honey in a jar, let it sit overnight.

- **How to Use:** Take 1-2 teaspoons of the syrup as needed.

- **Dosage:** As needed.

- **Side Effect:** May cause bad breath or digestive discomfort.

- **Precaution:** Avoid if allergic to onions.

14. **Horseradish Tincture:**

- **Definition:** Horseradish tincture is a potent decongestant that clears sinus congestion.

- **Ingredients:** Fresh horseradish root, apple cider vinegar.

- **How to Prepare:** Grate horseradish root and steep it in apple cider vinegar for 2-3 weeks, strain.

- **How to Use:** Take 1 teaspoon diluted in water.

- **Dosage:** 1-2 teaspoons per day.

- **Side Effect:** May cause stomach upset or irritation.

- **Precaution:** Avoid if pregnant or have gastrointestinal issues.

15. **Grapefruit Seed Extract Nasal Rinse:**

- **Definition:** Grapefruit seed extract nasal rinse helps clear nasal passages and reduce mucus buildup.

- **Ingredients:** Grapefruit seed extract, distilled water, saline solution.

- **How to Prepare:** Mix grapefruit seed extract with distilled water and saline solution.

- **How to Use:** Use a nasal rinse bottle to irrigate nasal passages.

- **Dosage:** Use as needed.

- **Side Effect:** May cause irritation or burning sensation in the nasal passages.

- **Precaution:** Ensure proper dilution to avoid irritation.

Practical Tips for Incorporation

When incorporating herbal teas and supplements into your cleanse regimen, consider the following practical tips:

1. **Choose High-Quality Products**: Select high-quality herbal teas and supplements from reputable brands to ensure purity, potency, and safety.

2. **Follow Dosage Recommendations**: Follow the dosage recommendations provided on the product labels or as recommended by a qualified healthcare professional. Start with a lower dose and gradually increase as needed.

3. **Stay Hydrated**: Drink plenty of water throughout the day to stay hydrated and support the body's natural detoxification processes.

4. **Listen to Your Body**: Pay attention to how your body responds to herbal teas and supplements. If you experience any adverse reactions or discomfort, discontinue use and consult with a healthcare professional.

5. **Incorporate Variety**: Experiment with different herbal teas and supplements to incorporate a variety of beneficial herbs and nutrients into your cleanse regimen.

6. **Combine with Lifestyle Modifications**: Herbal teas and supplements work best when combined with other lifestyle

modifications such as a healthy diet, regular exercise, stress management, and adequate sleep.

Conclusion

Incorporating herbal teas and supplements into your mucus cleanse regimen can enhance the effectiveness of the cleanse and support optimal results. Herbal teas containing mucolytic, expectorant, and anti-inflammatory herbs can help to reduce excess mucus and promote respiratory health, while detoxifying herbal supplements can support liver function, aid digestion, and eliminate toxins from the body. By choosing high-quality products, following dosage recommendations, staying hydrated, and listening to your body, you can maximize the benefits of herbal teas and supplements and enjoy improved well-being during your cleanse journey.

CHAPTER NINE

Managing Detox Symptoms and Supporting Your Body's Natural Processes

Embarking on a mucus cleanse or detoxification program can sometimes trigger temporary discomfort or symptoms as the body releases accumulated toxins and adjusts to dietary and lifestyle changes. It's essential to support your body's natural detoxification processes and manage any detox symptoms that may arise during the cleanse. In this guide, we'll explore strategies for managing detox symptoms and supporting your body's natural processes to promote a safe and effective cleanse experience.

Understanding Detox Symptoms

Detox symptoms can vary widely depending on individual factors such as the extent of toxin accumulation, overall health status, and the specific cleanse protocol being followed. Common detox symptoms may include:

1. **Fatigue**: As the body mobilizes toxins for elimination, individuals may experience temporary fatigue or lethargy.

2. **Headaches**: Detoxification can sometimes trigger headaches or migraines as the body releases toxins and adjusts to dietary changes.

3. **Digestive Disturbances**: Changes in diet and increased water intake may lead to temporary digestive discomfort such as bloating, gas, or diarrhea.

4. **Skin Breakouts**: Skin may temporarily worsen as the body eliminates toxins through the skin, leading to acne, rashes, or other skin eruptions.

5. **Flu-like Symptoms**: Some individuals may experience flu-like symptoms such as body aches, chills, and congestion as the body undergoes detoxification.

Strategies for Managing Detox Symptoms

While detox symptoms are typically temporary and a sign that the body is eliminating toxins, there are several strategies you can employ to manage discomfort and support your body's natural processes:

1. **Hydration**: Drink plenty of water throughout the day to support the body's detoxification processes and promote hydration. Herbal teas, lemon water, and electrolyte-rich drinks can also help to replenish fluids and support detoxification.

2. **Gentle Exercise**: Engage in gentle exercise such as walking, yoga, or stretching to support circulation, lymphatic drainage, and the elimination of toxins from the body. Avoid strenuous exercise that may exacerbate fatigue or discomfort.

3. **Rest and Relaxation**: Prioritize rest and relaxation to support the body's healing processes and reduce stress. Practice mindfulness meditation, deep breathing exercises, or take warm baths to promote relaxation and support detoxification.

4. **Nutrient-Rich Diet**: Eat a nutrient-rich diet that supports detoxification and provides essential vitamins, minerals, and antioxidants. Focus on whole foods such as fruits, vegetables, whole grains, lean proteins, and healthy fats to nourish your body and support optimal health.

5. **Herbal Support**: Incorporate herbal remedies such as ginger, peppermint, chamomile, or licorice root to support digestion, reduce inflammation, and alleviate detox symptoms. Herbal teas, tinctures, or supplements can provide targeted support during the cleanse process.

6. **Gradual Transition**: If transitioning to a new diet or cleanse protocol, gradually introduce dietary changes to minimize detox symptoms and support the body's adjustment process. Start by reducing processed foods, sugars, caffeine, and

alcohol, and gradually increase intake of whole foods, herbal teas, and supplements.

7. **Consultation with a Healthcare Professional**: If experiencing severe or prolonged detox symptoms, consult with a qualified healthcare professional for personalized guidance and recommendations. They can assess your individual health status, provide tailored support, and address any underlying issues that may be contributing to detox symptoms.

Supporting Your Body's Natural Processes

In addition to managing detox symptoms, it's essential to support your body's natural detoxification processes throughout the cleanse. Here are some strategies for promoting optimal detoxification and overall well-being:

1. **Liver Support**: Support liver function with herbs such as milk thistle, dandelion root, turmeric, and burdock root, which help to promote liver detoxification pathways and eliminate toxins from the body.

2. **Kidney Support**: Support kidney function with herbs such as nettle leaf, parsley, dandelion leaf, and corn silk, which help to promote kidney filtration and eliminate waste products from the body.

3. **Colon Support**: Support colon health and elimination with fiber-rich foods, hydrating beverages, and herbal remedies such as psyllium husk, flaxseed, aloe vera, and triphala, which help to promote bowel regularity and detoxification.

4. **Lymphatic Support**: Support lymphatic drainage and circulation with dry brushing, lymphatic massage, rebounding, and herbal remedies such as cleavers, red clover, calendula, and echinacea, which help to promote lymphatic flow and detoxification.

5. **Skin Support**: Support skin health and detoxification with regular exfoliation, sweating through exercise or sauna sessions, and herbal remedies such as burdock root, red clover, cleavers, and calendula, which help to promote skin detoxification and clarity.

Conclusion

Managing detox symptoms and supporting your body's natural processes are essential aspects of a safe and effective cleanse experience. By staying hydrated, engaging in gentle exercise, prioritizing rest and relaxation, eating a nutrient-rich diet, incorporating herbal support, and consulting with a healthcare professional as needed, you can navigate detoxification with confidence and promote optimal well-being. With mindful attention and self-care, you can support your body's natural detoxification processes and enjoy the benefits of a mucus cleanse or detoxification program.

CHAPTER TEN

Post-Cleanse Maintenance: Lifestyle Tips for Long-Term Mucus Reduction and Health

Completing a mucus cleanse or detoxification program is an important step towards improving respiratory health, supporting immune function, and promoting overall well-being. However, maintaining the benefits of the cleanse and preventing the recurrence of excess mucus requires ongoing attention to lifestyle factors that influence health. In this guide, we'll explore lifestyle tips for long-term mucus reduction and health maintenance, including dietary recommendations, stress management strategies, environmental considerations, and supportive practices for respiratory and immune health.

1. Maintain a Healthy Diet

A nutrient-rich diet is essential for long-term mucus reduction and overall health. Focus on whole, unprocessed foods that support respiratory health, reduce inflammation, and promote immune function. Incorporate plenty of fruits, vegetables, whole grains, lean proteins, and healthy fats into your daily meals. Minimize or eliminate inflammatory foods such as processed foods, refined sugars, trans fats, and excessive dairy products, which can contribute to mucus production and inflammation.

2. Stay Hydrated

Adequate hydration is crucial for maintaining optimal mucus viscosity and supporting mucociliary clearance in the respiratory tract. Drink plenty of water throughout the day to keep mucous membranes moist and promote the elimination of toxins from the body. Herbal teas, broths, and fresh juices can also contribute to hydration and provide additional benefits for respiratory and immune health.

3. Support Digestive Health

Gut health plays a significant role in overall immunity and mucus reduction. Incorporate fiber-rich foods such as fruits, vegetables, whole grains, and legumes into your diet to support digestive function and promote regular bowel movements. Probiotic-rich foods such as yogurt, kefir, sauerkraut, and kimchi can also help to maintain a healthy balance of gut bacteria and support immune function.

4. Manage Stress

Chronic stress can weaken the immune system, exacerbate inflammation, and contribute to mucus-related symptoms. Practice stress management techniques such as meditation, deep breathing exercises, yoga, tai chi, or mindfulness practices to promote relaxation, reduce stress hormones, and support overall well-being. Prioritize self-care activities that nourish your mind, body, and spirit, such as spending time in nature, journaling, or engaging in hobbies you enjoy.

5. Maintain Respiratory Hygiene

Good respiratory hygiene is essential for preventing respiratory infections and reducing mucus production. Practice regular handwashing, avoid touching your face, and cover your mouth and nose when coughing or sneezing to prevent the spread of germs. Use saline nasal sprays or neti pots to irrigate the nasal passages and remove allergens, irritants, and excess mucus. Keep indoor air clean and well-ventilated, and avoid exposure to environmental pollutants, cigarette smoke, and other respiratory irritants.

6. Exercise Regularly

Regular exercise supports immune function, enhances circulation, and promotes respiratory health. Engage in aerobic exercise, strength training, or flexibility exercises such as walking, jogging, swimming, cycling, yoga, or tai chi to support mucus reduction and overall well-being. Aim for at least 30 minutes of moderate-intensity exercise most days of the week, and incorporate activities that you enjoy and that fit your fitness level and preferences.

7. Get Adequate Sleep

Quality sleep is essential for immune function, stress management, and overall health. Aim for 7-9 hours of restorative sleep each night to support mucus reduction, tissue repair, and detoxification processes. Create a relaxing bedtime routine, optimize your sleep environment by keeping it cool, dark, and quiet, and avoid stimulants such as caffeine and electronics before bedtime. If you struggle with sleep, consider practicing relaxation techniques, such as meditation or deep breathing exercises, to promote restful sleep.

8. Seek Regular Healthcare

Regular healthcare visits are essential for monitoring your health, addressing any underlying issues, and preventing recurrent mucus-related symptoms. Schedule regular check-ups with your healthcare provider, particularly if you have chronic respiratory conditions such as asthma, allergies, or sinusitis. Discuss any changes in your symptoms, lifestyle habits, or medication regimen with your healthcare provider, and follow their recommendations for optimal health and well-being.

Conclusion

Maintaining the benefits of a mucus cleanse and supporting long-term health requires attention to various lifestyle factors that influence respiratory health, immune function, and overall well-being. By incorporating healthy dietary habits, stress management strategies, respiratory hygiene practices, regular exercise, adequate sleep, and regular healthcare visits into your routine, you can promote mucus reduction and enjoy sustained health and vitality. With mindful attention and consistent self-care, you can support your body's natural healing processes and thrive in the long term.

BONUS: SOME HOLISTIC APPROACHES TO KNOW

Herban Iron:

Definition: Herban Iron is a dietary supplement designed to provide an easily absorbable form of iron to support healthy iron levels in the body. It's particularly beneficial for individuals with iron deficiency or anemia.

Ingredients: Herban Iron typically contains iron in the form of ferrous bisglycinate, which is a highly bioavailable and gentle form of iron that is less likely to cause digestive upset or constipation compared to other forms of iron. It may also contain other ingredients such as vitamin C to enhance iron absorption.

How to Prepare: Herban Iron is usually available in capsule or liquid form. Capsules are taken orally with water, while liquid forms may be mixed with water or juice before consumption. It's important to follow the recommended dosage on the product label.

Dosage: The appropriate dosage of Herban Iron depends on factors such as age, gender, and the severity of iron deficiency. It's important to consult with a healthcare professional to determine the correct dosage for individual needs.

How to Use: Herban Iron capsules are typically taken orally with water, while liquid forms may be mixed with water or juice before consumption. It's important to take Herban Iron as directed and to avoid taking it with dairy products, antacids, or other substances that may interfere with iron absorption.

Side Effects: While Herban Iron is generally considered safe for most people when used as directed, some individuals may experience mild side effects such as gastrointestinal discomfort or constipation. It's important to consult with a healthcare professional before starting any new supplement regimen, especially if you have underlying health conditions or are taking medications.

Hydrangea:

Definition: Hydrangea, scientifically known as Hydrangea arborescens, is a flowering shrub native to North America. It has been used traditionally in herbal medicine for its potential diuretic and anti-inflammatory properties.

Ingredients: Hydrangea contains several bioactive compounds, including saponins, flavonoids, and glycosides. These compounds are believed to contribute to the herb's medicinal properties, including its potential as a diuretic, kidney tonic, and anti-inflammatory agent.

How to Prepare: Hydrangea root is typically prepared and consumed as an herbal tea or tincture. To make tea, dried hydrangea root is steeped in hot water for several minutes before being strained and consumed. Tinctures are prepared by steeping the root in alcohol or vinegar to extract its active compounds.

Dosage: The appropriate dosage of hydrangea can vary depending on factors such as age, health status, and the specific preparation being used. It's important to follow the recommended dosage on the product label or consult with a qualified herbalist or healthcare professional for personalized guidance.

How to Use: Hydrangea tea or tincture is typically taken orally. It's important to use hydrangea products as directed and to discontinue use if any adverse effects occur.

Side Effects: Hydrangea is generally considered safe for most people when used in moderate amounts. However, some individuals may experience digestive upset or allergic reactions. It may also interact with certain medications or have adverse effects in individuals with certain health conditions. It's important to use hydrangea under the guidance of a healthcare professional and to discontinue use if any adverse effects occur.

Irish Moss:

Definition: Irish Moss, scientifically known as Chondrus crispus, is a species of red algae or seaweed native to the Atlantic coastlines of Europe and North America. It has been used for centuries in traditional Irish and Scottish cuisine, as well as in herbal medicine.

Ingredients: Irish Moss is rich in various nutrients, including iodine, sulfur compounds, vitamins (such as vitamin A, vitamin K, and vitamin B12), minerals (including calcium, magnesium, potassium, and sodium), and polysaccharides (such as carrageenan). These nutrients are believed to contribute to the herb's potential health benefits.

How to Prepare: Irish Moss is typically prepared by soaking it in water to rehydrate and soften it before use. It can be added to soups, stews, smoothies, desserts, and other dishes as a thickening agent or nutritional supplement.

Dosage: The appropriate dosage of Irish Moss can vary depending on factors such as age, health status, and the specific preparation being used. It's important to follow recipes or guidelines for culinary use and to consult with a healthcare professional for guidance on using Irish Moss as a dietary supplement.

How to Use: Irish Moss can be used in culinary applications to add thickness and nutritional value to dishes. It can also be consumed as a dietary supplement in the form of capsules, powders, or extracts.

Side Effects: Irish Moss is generally considered safe for most people when consumed in moderate amounts as part of a balanced diet. However, some individuals may be allergic to seaweed or carrageenan, a compound found in Irish Moss that is used as a food additive. It's important to discontinue use if any adverse effects occur and to consult with a healthcare professional if you have any concerns.

Irish Sea Moss:

Definition: Irish Sea Moss is a term often used interchangeably with Irish Moss, referring to the same species of red algae, Chondrus crispus. It's harvested from the rocky shores of the Atlantic coastlines of Europe and North America.

Ingredients: Irish Sea Moss shares the same nutritional profile as Irish Moss, containing iodine, vitamins, minerals, and polysaccharides. It's valued for its potential health benefits, including supporting thyroid function, boosting immune health, and promoting digestion.

How to Prepare: Irish Sea Moss is prepared in the same way as Irish Moss, by soaking it in water to rehydrate and soften it before use. It can be used in culinary applications or consumed as a dietary supplement.

Dosage: The dosage of Irish Sea Moss depends on the form and intended use. As a dietary supplement, it's important to follow the recommended dosage on the product label or consult with a healthcare professional for personalized guidance.

How to Use: Irish Sea Moss can be used in various culinary applications, including soups, smoothies, desserts, and sauces. It can also be consumed as a dietary supplement in the form of capsules, powders, or extracts.

Side Effects: Similar to Irish Moss, Irish Sea Moss is generally considered safe for most people when consumed in moderate amounts. However, individuals with seaweed allergies or sensitivities to carrageenan should exercise caution. It's important to discontinue use if any adverse effects occur and to consult with a healthcare professional if you have any concerns.

Lymphalin:

Definition: Lymphalin is a herbal supplement formulated to support lymphatic system health. The lymphatic system plays a crucial role in immune function and waste removal in the body, and Lymphalin is designed to promote its proper function.

Ingredients: Lymphalin typically contains a blend of herbs and botanical extracts known for their traditional use in supporting lymphatic system health. Common ingredients may include cleavers, red clover, echinacea, burdock root, and calendula, among others.

How to Prepare: Lymphalin is usually available in capsule or liquid form. Capsules are taken orally with water, while liquid forms may be mixed with water or juice before consumption. It's important to follow the recommended dosage on the product label.

Dosage: The appropriate dosage of Lymphalin can vary depending on the specific product and individual needs. It's important to follow the recommended dosage on the product label or consult with a healthcare professional for personalized guidance.

How to Use: Lymphalin capsules are typically taken orally with water, while liquid forms may be mixed with water or juice before consumption. It's often recommended to take Lymphalin on an empty stomach for optimal absorption.

Side Effects: Lymphalin is generally considered safe for most people when used as directed. However, some individuals may experience mild side effects such as gastrointestinal discomfort or allergic reactions to certain ingredients. It's important to consult with a healthcare provider before starting any new supplement regimen, especially if you have underlying health conditions or are taking medications.

Manjakani:

Definition: Manjakani, also known as Quercus infectoria or oak gall, is a natural substance derived from the oak tree. It has been used for centuries in traditional medicine for its potential health benefits, particularly for women's health and vaginal tightening.

Ingredients: Manjakani contains various bioactive compounds, including tannins, flavonoids, and gallic acid. These compounds are believed to contribute to the herb's medicinal properties, including its potential as an astringent and antiseptic agent.

How to Prepare: Manjakani is typically available in powder, capsule, or liquid extract form. It can be taken orally or used topically depending on the intended use. For vaginal tightening, manjakani may be applied topically as a gel or inserted into the vagina in capsule form.

Dosage: The appropriate dosage of manjakani can vary depending on factors such as age, health status, and the specific preparation being used. It's important to follow the recommended dosage on the product label or consult with a qualified herbalist or healthcare professional for personalized guidance.

How to Use: Manjakani can be taken orally or used topically depending on the intended use. It's important to use manjakani products as directed and to discontinue use if any adverse effects occur.

Side Effects: Manjakani is generally considered safe for most people when used in moderate amounts. However, some individuals may experience allergic reactions or skin irritation when used topically. It's important to use manjakani under the guidance of a healthcare professional and to discontinue use if any adverse effects occur.

Red Clover:

Definition: Red clover, scientifically known as Trifolium pratense, is a flowering plant belonging to the legume family. It's native to Europe, Western Asia, and Northwest Africa but has been naturalized in many other regions. Red clover has been used in traditional medicine for various purposes, including its potential to support women's health and menopausal symptoms.

Ingredients: Red clover contains several bioactive compounds, including isoflavones (such as genistein and daidzein), flavonoids, and phytoestrogens. These compounds are believed to contribute to the herb's medicinal properties, including its potential as a hormone-balancing agent and its ability to support cardiovascular health.

How to Prepare: Red clover is typically prepared and consumed as an herbal tea or tincture. To make tea, dried red clover flowers are steeped in hot water for several minutes before being strained and consumed. Tinctures are prepared by steeping the flowers in alcohol or vinegar to extract their active compounds.

Dosage: The appropriate dosage of red clover can vary depending on factors such as age, health status, and the specific preparation being used. It's important to follow the recommended dosage on the product label or consult with a qualified herbalist or healthcare professional for personalized guidance.

How to Use: Red clover tea or tincture is typically taken orally. It's important to use red clover products as directed and to discontinue use if any adverse effects occur.

Side Effects: Red clover is generally considered safe for most people when used in moderate amounts. However, some individuals may experience allergic reactions or digestive upset. It may also interact with certain medications or have adverse effects in individuals with certain health conditions. It's important to use red clover under the guidance of a healthcare professional and to discontinue use if any adverse effects occur.

Red Raspberry:

Definition: Red raspberry, scientifically known as Rubus idaeus, is a species of raspberry native to Europe and northern Asia. It's widely cultivated for its delicious berries and has been used in traditional medicine for various purposes, including its potential to support women's health during pregnancy and childbirth.

Ingredients: Red raspberry contains several bioactive compounds, including flavonoids, ellagic acid, anthocyanins, and vitamin C.

These compounds are believed to contribute to the herb's medicinal properties, including its potential as an antioxidant, anti-inflammatory, and uterine tonic.

How to Prepare: Red raspberry leaf is typically prepared and consumed as an herbal tea or infusion. To make tea, dried red raspberry leaves are steeped in hot water for several minutes before being strained and consumed.

Dosage: The appropriate dosage of red raspberry leaf can vary depending on factors such as age, health status, and the specific preparation being used. It's important to follow the recommended dosage on the product label or consult with a qualified herbalist or healthcare professional for personalized guidance.

How to Use: Red raspberry leaf tea is typically taken orally. It's often recommended for pregnant individuals in the later stages of pregnancy to support uterine health and prepare for childbirth. It's important to use red raspberry leaf products as directed and to discontinue use if any adverse effects occur.

Side Effects: Red raspberry leaf is generally considered safe for most people when used in moderate amounts. However, some individuals may experience allergic reactions or digestive upset. Pregnant individuals should consult with a healthcare professional before using red raspberry leaf, especially if they have any underlying health conditions or are taking medications.

It's important to use red raspberry leaf under the guidance of a healthcare professional and to discontinue use if any adverse effects occur.

Tila:

Definition: Tila, also known as linden flower or lime blossom, refers to the flowers of the Tilia genus, primarily Tilia europaea and Tilia cordata. These trees are native to Europe, but they are also cultivated in other regions for their fragrant and medicinal flowers.

Ingredients: Tila flowers contain various bioactive compounds, including flavonoids, phenolic acids, and volatile oils. These compounds are believed to contribute to the herb's medicinal properties, including its potential as a mild sedative, anxiolytic, and anti-inflammatory agent.

How to Prepare: Tila flowers are typically prepared and consumed as an herbal tea or infusion. To make tea, dried tila flowers are steeped in hot water for several minutes before being strained and consumed.

Dosage: The appropriate dosage of tila can vary depending on factors such as age, health status, and the specific preparation being used. It's important to follow the recommended dosage on the product label or consult with a qualified herbalist or healthcare professional for personalized guidance.

How to Use: Tila tea is typically taken orally. It's often consumed in the evening as a calming bedtime beverage or during times of stress or anxiety. It's important to use tila products as directed and to discontinue use if any adverse effects occur.

Side Effects: Tila is generally considered safe for most people when used in moderate amounts. However, some individuals may experience allergic reactions or digestive upset. It may also interact with certain medications or have adverse effects in individuals with certain health conditions. It's important to use tila under the guidance of a healthcare professional and to discontinue use if any adverse effects occur.

Valerian:

Definition: Valerian, scientifically known as Valeriana officinalis, is a perennial flowering plant native to Europe and Asia. It has been used for centuries in traditional medicine for its potential calming and sedative effects.

Ingredients: Valerian root contains several bioactive compounds, including valerenic acid, valepotriates, and volatile oils. These compounds are believed to contribute to the herb's medicinal properties, including its potential as a sedative, anxiolytic, and sleep aid.

How to Prepare: Valerian root is typically prepared and consumed as an herbal tea, tincture, or capsule. To make tea, dried valerian root is steeped in hot water for several minutes before being strained and consumed. Tinctures are prepared by steeping the root in alcohol or vinegar to extract its active compounds.

Dosage: The appropriate dosage of valerian can vary depending on factors such as age, health status, and the specific preparation being used. It's important to follow the recommended dosage on the product label or consult with a qualified herbalist or healthcare professional for personalized guidance.

How to Use: Valerian tea, tincture, or capsules are typically taken orally. It's often consumed in the evening as a sleep aid or during times of stress or anxiety. It's important to use valerian products as directed and to discontinue use if any adverse effects occur.

Side Effects: Valerian is generally considered safe for most people when used in moderate amounts. However, some individuals may experience mild side effects such as drowsiness, headache, or gastrointestinal upset. It may also interact with certain medications or have adverse effects in individuals with certain health conditions. It's important to use valerian under the guidance of a healthcare professional and to discontinue use if any adverse effects occur.

Wild Cherry Bark:

Definition: Wild cherry bark, scientifically known as Prunus serotina, is the bark obtained from the black cherry tree native to North America. It has been used traditionally in Native American and folk medicine for its potential health benefits, particularly for respiratory and digestive issues.

Ingredients: Wild cherry bark contains various bioactive compounds, including cyanogenic glycosides (such as prunasin and amygdalin), flavonoids, and phenolic acids. These compounds are believed to contribute to the herb's medicinal properties, including its potential as an expectorant, cough suppressant, and mild sedative.

How to Prepare: Wild cherry bark is typically prepared and consumed as an herbal tea, decoction, or syrup. To make tea, dried wild cherry bark is steeped in hot water for several minutes before being strained and consumed. Decoctions involve boiling the bark in water to extract its active compounds, while syrups are made by simmering the bark with sugar or honey to create a thick, sweet liquid.

Dosage: The appropriate dosage of wild cherry bark can vary depending on factors such as age, health status, and the specific preparation being used. It's important to follow the recommended dosage on the product label or consult with a qualified herbalist or healthcare professional for personalized guidance.

How to Use: Wild cherry bark tea, decoction, or syrup is typically taken orally. It's often consumed to soothe coughs, sore throats, and other respiratory symptoms. It's important to use wild cherry bark products as directed and to discontinue use if any adverse effects occur.

Side Effects: Wild cherry bark is generally considered safe for most people when used in moderate amounts. However, it contains cyanogenic glycosides, which can release cyanide in the body when metabolized. While the risk of cyanide poisoning from consuming wild cherry bark is low when used appropriately, excessive intake or prolonged use may lead to adverse effects. It's important to use wild cherry bark under the guidance of a healthcare professional and to discontinue use if any adverse effects occur.

Yellowdock:

Definition: Yellowdock, scientifically known as Rumex crispus, is a perennial flowering plant native to Europe and western Asia but is also found in North America. It has a long history of use in traditional medicine, particularly among Indigenous peoples, for its potential health benefits.

Ingredients: Yellowdock root contains various bioactive compounds, including anthraquinone glycosides (such as emodin and chrysophanol), tannins, and vitamins (including vitamin A and vitamin C). These compounds are believed to contribute to the herb's medicinal properties, including its potential as a laxative, blood cleanser, and liver tonic.

How to Prepare: Yellowdock root is typically prepared and consumed as an herbal tea, tincture, or capsule. To make tea, dried yellowdock root is steeped in hot water for several minutes before being strained and consumed. Tinctures are prepared by steeping the root in alcohol or vinegar to extract its active compounds.

Dosage: The appropriate dosage of yellowdock can vary depending on factors such as age, health status, and the specific preparation being used. It's important to follow the recommended dosage on the product label or consult with a qualified herbalist or healthcare professional for personalized guidance.

How to Use: Yellowdock tea, tincture, or capsules are typically taken orally. It's often consumed to support digestion, promote bowel regularity, and cleanse the blood. It's important to use yellowdock products as directed and to discontinue use if any adverse effects occur.

Side Effects: Yellowdock is generally considered safe for most people when used in moderate amounts. However, some individuals may experience mild side effects such as gastrointestinal upset or allergic reactions. It may also interact with certain medications or have adverse effects in individuals with certain health conditions. It's important to use yellowdock under the guidance of a healthcare professional and to discontinue use if any adverse effects occur.

Yellowdock Root:

Definition: Yellowdock root, scientifically known as Rumex crispus, is the root of a perennial flowering plant native to Europe and western Asia, also found in North America. It has a long history of use in traditional medicine, particularly among Indigenous peoples, for its potential health benefits.

Ingredients: Yellowdock root contains various bioactive compounds, including anthraquinone glycosides (such as emodin and chrysophanol), tannins, and vitamins (including vitamin A and vitamin C). These compounds are believed to contribute to the herb's medicinal properties, including its potential as a laxative, blood cleanser, and liver tonic.

How to Prepare: Yellowdock root is typically prepared and consumed as an herbal tea, tincture, or capsule. To make tea, dried yellowdock root is steeped in hot water for several minutes before being strained and consumed. Tinctures are prepared by steeping the root in alcohol or vinegar to extract its active compounds.

Dosage: The appropriate dosage of yellowdock root can vary depending on factors such as age, health status, and the specific preparation being used. It's important to follow the recommended dosage on the product label or consult with a qualified herbalist or healthcare professional for personalized guidance.

How to Use: Yellowdock root tea, tincture, or capsules are typically taken orally. It's often consumed to support digestion, promote bowel regularity, and cleanse the blood. It's important to use yellowdock root products as directed and to discontinue use if any adverse effects occur.

Side Effects: Yellowdock root is generally considered safe for most people when used in moderate amounts. However, some individuals may experience mild side effects such as gastrointestinal upset or allergic reactions. It may also interact with certain medications or have adverse effects in individuals with certain health conditions. It's important to use yellowdock root under the guidance of a healthcare professional and to discontinue use if any adverse effects occur.

Agrimony:

Definition: Agrimony, scientifically known as Agrimonia eupatoria, is a perennial herbaceous plant native to Europe, Asia, and North America. It has a long history of use in traditional medicine, particularly in European folk medicine, for its potential health benefits.

Ingredients: Agrimony contains various bioactive compounds, including tannins, flavonoids, phenolic acids, and volatile oils. These compounds are believed to contribute to the herb's medicinal properties, including its potential as an astringent, anti-inflammatory, and digestive aid.

How to Prepare: Agrimony is typically prepared and consumed as an herbal tea, tincture, or poultice. To make tea, dried agrimony leaves and flowers are steeped in hot water for several minutes before being strained and consumed. Tinctures are prepared by steeping the herb in alcohol or vinegar to extract its active compounds.

Dosage: The appropriate dosage of agrimony can vary depending on factors such as age, health status, and the specific preparation being used. It's important to follow the recommended dosage on the product label or consult with a qualified herbalist or healthcare professional for personalized guidance.

How to Use: Agrimony tea, tincture, or poultice is typically taken orally or applied topically. It's often consumed to soothe gastrointestinal issues, such as indigestion and diarrhea, or used externally to treat skin conditions.

Side Effects: Agrimony is generally considered safe for most people when used in moderate amounts. However, some individuals may experience allergic reactions or gastrointestinal upset. It may also interact with certain medications or have adverse effects in individuals with certain health conditions. It's important to use agrimony under the guidance of a healthcare professional and to discontinue use if any adverse effects occur.

Alfalfa:

Definition: Alfalfa, scientifically known as Medicago sativa, is a flowering plant in the pea family native to Asia but cultivated worldwide. It's primarily grown as fodder for livestock, but it has also been used in traditional medicine for its potential health benefits.

Ingredients: Alfalfa contains various bioactive compounds, including vitamins (such as vitamin A, vitamin C, and vitamin K), minerals (including calcium, magnesium, and potassium), amino acids, and phytoestrogens. These compounds are believed to contribute to the herb's medicinal properties, including its potential as a nutritive tonic, diuretic, and hormone balancer.

How to Prepare: Alfalfa is typically consumed as sprouts, herbal tea, or in supplement form (such as capsules or tablets). To make tea, dried alfalfa leaves are steeped in hot water for several minutes before being strained and consumed.

Dosage: The appropriate dosage of alfalfa can vary depending on factors such as age, health status, and the specific preparation being used. It's important to follow the recommended dosage on the product label or consult with a qualified herbalist or healthcare professional for personalized guidance.

How to Use: Alfalfa sprouts, tea, or supplements are typically taken orally. It's often consumed as a dietary supplement to support overall health and well-being, as well as to promote kidney health and hormone balance.

Side Effects: Alfalfa is generally considered safe for most people when consumed in moderate amounts. However, some individuals may experience allergic reactions or digestive upset. It may also interact with certain medications or have adverse effects in individuals with certain health conditions, such as autoimmune diseases or hormone-sensitive conditions. Pregnant or breastfeeding individuals should consult with a healthcare professional before using alfalfa supplements. It's important to use alfalfa under the guidance of a healthcare professional and to discontinue use if any adverse effects occur.

Ashwagandha:

Definition: Ashwagandha, scientifically known as Withaniasomnifera, is a small shrub native to India, the Middle East, and parts of Africa. It has a long history of use in Ayurvedic medicine for its potential health benefits, particularly for its adaptogenic properties.

Ingredients: Ashwagandha root contains various bioactive compounds, including alkaloids (such as withanolides), steroidal lactones, and flavonoids. These compounds are believed to contribute to the herb's medicinal properties, including its potential as an adaptogen, anti-inflammatory, and immune-modulating agent.

How to Prepare: Ashwagandha is typically consumed as a powdered root, herbal tea, tincture, or in supplement form (such as capsules or tablets). To make tea, dried ashwagandha root is steeped in hot water for several minutes before being strained and consumed.

Dosage: The appropriate dosage of ashwagandha can vary depending on factors such as age, health status, and the specific preparation being used. It's important to follow the recommended dosage on the product label or consult with a qualified herbalist or healthcare professional for personalized guidance.

How to Use: Ashwagandha powder, tea, tincture, or supplements are typically taken orally. It's often consumed to support stress management, promote relaxation, and boost overall vitality and well-being.

Side Effects: Ashwagandha is generally considered safe for most people when used in moderate amounts. However, some individuals may experience mild side effects such as gastrointestinal upset or drowsiness. It may also interact with certain medications or have adverse effects in individuals with certain health conditions, such as autoimmune diseases or thyroid disorders. Pregnant or breastfeeding individuals should consult with a healthcare professional before using ashwagandha supplements. It's important to use ashwagandha under the guidance of a healthcare professional and to discontinue use if any adverse effects occur.

Astragalus:

Definition: Astragalus, scientifically known as Astragalus membranaceus, is a flowering plant native to China and Mongolia but also found in other parts of Asia. It has been used for centuries in traditional Chinese medicine for its potential health benefits, particularly for its immune-enhancing properties.

Ingredients: Astragalus root contains various bioactive compounds, including polysaccharides, saponins (such as astragalosides), flavonoids, and amino acids. These compounds are believed to contribute to the herb's medicinal properties, including its potential as an adaptogen, immunomodulator, and anti-inflammatory agent.

How to Prepare: Astragalus is typically consumed as a powdered root, herbal tea, tincture, or in supplement form (such as capsules or tablets). To make tea, dried astragalus root slices are simmered in water for several minutes before being strained and consumed.

Dosage: The appropriate dosage of astragalus can vary depending on factors such as age, health status, and the specific preparation being used. It's important to follow the recommended dosage on the product label or consult with a qualified herbalist or healthcare professional for personalized guidance.

How to Use: Astragalus powder, tea, tincture, or supplements are typically taken orally. It's often consumed to support immune function, promote vitality, and enhance overall well-being.

Side Effects: Astragalus is generally considered safe for most people when used in moderate amounts. However, some individuals may experience mild side effects such as gastrointestinal upset or allergic reactions. It may also interact with certain medications or have adverse effects in individuals with certain health conditions, such as autoimmune diseases or diabetes. Pregnant or breastfeeding individuals should consult with a healthcare professional before using astragalus supplements. It's important to use astragalus under the guidance of a healthcare professional and to discontinue use if any adverse effects occur.

Sarsaparilla:

Definition: Sarsaparilla refers to several species of plants belonging to the Smilax genus, including Smilax regelii and Smilax officinalis. It has been used historically in traditional medicine for its potential health benefits, particularly for its purported detoxifying and anti-inflammatory properties.

Ingredients: Sarsaparilla contains various bioactive compounds, including saponins (such as sarsaponin and smilagenin), flavonoids, phenolic acids, and sterols. These compounds are believed to contribute to the herb's medicinal properties, including its potential as a diuretic, blood purifier, and anti-inflammatory agent.

How to Prepare: Sarsaparilla root is typically prepared and consumed as an herbal tea, decoction, or tincture. To make tea, dried sarsaparilla root is steeped in hot water for several minutes before being strained and consumed. Decoctions involve boiling the root in water to extract its active compounds, while tinctures are prepared by steeping the root in alcohol or vinegar.

Dosage: The appropriate dosage of sarsaparilla can vary depending on factors such as age, health status, and the specific preparation being used. It's important to follow the recommended dosage on the product label or consult with a qualified herbalist or healthcare professional for personalized guidance.

How to Use: Sarsaparilla tea or tincture is typically taken orally. It's important to use sarsaparilla products as directed and to discontinue use if any adverse effects occur.

Side Effects: Sarsaparilla is generally considered safe for most people when used in moderate amounts. However, some individuals may experience allergic reactions or digestive upset. It may also interact with certain medications or have adverse effects in individuals with certain health conditions. It's important to use sarsaparilla under the guidance of a healthcare professional and to discontinue use if any adverse effects occur.

THE END